Considerations for Ensuring Safety and Efficacy of Vaccines and Therapeutic Proteins Manufactured by Using Platform Approaches

Summary of a Workshop

I0803810

Jeffrey Fox, Marilee Shelton-Davenport, and India Hook-Barnard, *Rapporteurs*

Board on Life Sciences

Division on Earth and Life Studies

NATIONAL RESEARCH COUNCIL
OF THE NATIONAL ACADEMIES

THE NATIONAL ACADEMIES PRESS
Washington, DC
www.nap.edu

THE NATIONAL ACADEMIES PRESS 500 Fifth Street, NW, Washington, DC 20001

NOTICE: The project that is the subject of this report was approved by the Governing Board of the National Research Council, whose members are drawn from the councils of the National Academy of Sciences, the National Academy of Engineering, and the Institute of Medicine. The members of the committee responsible for the report were chosen for their special competences and with regard for appropriate balance.

This study was supported by Contract W911NF-07-C-0081between the National Academy of Sciences and Department of the Army. Any opinions, findings, conclusions, or recommendations expressed in this publication are those of the authors and do not necessarily reflect the views of the organizations or agencies that provided support for the project.

International Standard Book Number - 13: 978-0-309-15321-8
International Standard Book Number - 10: 0-309-15321-2

Additional copies of this report are available from:

The National Academies Press
500 Fifth Street, NW
Lockbox 285
Washington, DC 20055

(800) 624-6242 or
(202) 334-3313 (in the Washington metropolitan area)
http://www.nap.edu

Copyright 2010 by the National Academy of Sciences. All rights reserved.

Printed in the United States of America

THE NATIONAL ACADEMIES

Advisers to the Nation on Science, Engineering, and Medicine

The **National Academy of Sciences** is a private, nonprofit, self-perpetuating society of distinguished scholars engaged in scientific and engineering research, dedicated to the furtherance of science and technology and to their use for the general welfare. Upon the authority of the charter granted to it by the Congress in 1863, the Academy has a mandate that requires it to advise the federal government on scientific and technical matters. Dr. Ralph J. Cicerone is president of the National Academy of Sciences.

The **National Academy of Engineering** was established in 1964, under the charter of the National Academy of Sciences, as a parallel organization of outstanding engineers. It is autonomous in its administration and in the selection of its members, sharing with the National Academy of Sciences the responsibility for advising the federal government. The National Academy of Engineering also sponsors engineering programs aimed at meeting national needs, encourages education and research, and recognizes the superior achievements of engineers. Dr. Charles M. Vest is president of the National Academy of Engineering.

The **Institute of Medicine** was established in 1970 by the National Academy of Sciences to secure the services of eminent members of appropriate professions in the examination of policy matters pertaining to the health of the public. The Institute acts under the responsibility given to the National Academy of Sciences by its congressional charter to be an adviser to the federal government and, upon its own initiative, to identify issues of medical care, research, and education. Dr. Harvey V. Fineberg is president of the Institute of Medicine.

The **National Research Council** was organized by the National Academy of Sciences in 1916 to associate the broad community of science and technology with the Academy's purposes of furthering knowledge and advising the federal government. Functioning in accordance with general policies determined by the Academy, the Council has become the principal operating agency of both the National Academy of Sciences and the National Academy of Engineering in providing services to the government, the public, and the scientific and engineering communities. The Council is administered jointly by both Academies and the Institute of Medicine. Dr. Ralph J. Cicerone and Dr. Charles M. Vest are chair and vice chair, respectively, of the National Research Council.

www.national-academies.org

NATIONAL RESEARCH COUNCIL STANDING COMMITTEE ON BIODEFENSE AT THE US DEPARTMENT OF DEFENSE

JENNIE HUNTER-CEVERA (Chair), RTI International, Research Triangle Park, NC
L. GARRY ADAMS, Texas A&M University, College Station, TX
JOHN F. ALDERETE, Washington State University, Pullman, WA
EDWARD J. ARCURI, Novartis Vaccines and Diagnostics, Inc., Cambridge, MA
MICHAEL ASCHER, University of California, Davis, CA
LESLIE BENET, University of California, San Francisco, CA
PHILIP E. COYLE III, Science Strategies, Sacramento, CA
STEPHEN W. DREW, Drew Solutions and Science Partners, LLC, Summit, NJ
DENISE FAUSTMAN, Harvard Medical School, Massachusetts General Hospital, Charlestown, MA
HARRY GREENBERG, Stanford University, Stanford, CA
CHARLES HOBBS, Lovelace Respiratory Research Institute, Albuquerque, NM
THOMAS INGLESBY, University of Pittsburgh Medical Center, Baltimore, MD
JAMES A. MARKS, University of California, San Francisco, CA
TIMOTHY MOSHIER, Syracuse Research Corporation, North Syracuse, NY
FRED MURPHY, University of Texas Medical Branch, Galveston, TX
KAREN NELSON, J. Craig Venter Institute, Rockville, MD
PETER A. PATRIARCA, Biologics Consulting Group, Inc., Bethesda, MD
JOHN A. SMITH, University of Alabama, Birmingham, AL
JIM SWEARENGEN, National Biodefense Analysis and Countermeasures Center, Frederick, MD
GRIFFIN TROTTER, Saint Louis University Center for Health Care Ethics, St. Louis, MO
DAVID H. WALKER, University of Texas Medical Branch, Galveston, TX

Staff

MARILEE K. SHELTON-DAVENPORT, Study Director
INDIA HOOK-BARNARD, Program Officer
REBECCA L. WALTER, Senior Program Assistant
NORMAN GROSSBLATT, Senior Editor
AMANDA L. MAZZAWI, Program Assistant

Sponsor

DEPARTMENT OF DEFENSE TRANSFORMATIONAL MEDICAL TECHNOLOGIES INITIATIVE

PLANNING GROUP FOR THE WORKSHOP ON CONSIDERATIONS FOR ENSURING SAFETY AND EFFICACY OF VACCINES AND THERAPEUTIC PROTEINS MANUFACTURED BY USING PLATFORM APPROACHES

JENNIE HUNTER-CEVERA (Chair), RTI International, Research Triangle Park, NC
EDWARD J. ARCURI, Novartis Vaccines and Diagnostics, Inc., Cambridge, MA
STEPHEN W. DREW, Drew Solutions and Science Partners, LLC, Summit, NJ
PETER A. PATRIARCA, Biologics Consulting Group, Inc., Bethesda, MD

Staff

MARILEE K. SHELTON-DAVENPORT, Study Director
INDIA HOOK-BARNARD, Program Officer
REBECCA L. WALTER, Senior Program Assistant

BOARD ON LIFE SCIENCES

Members

KEITH R. YAMAMOTO (Chair), University of California, San Francisco, CA
ANN M. ARVIN, Stanford University School of Medicine, Stanford, CA
BONNIE L. BASSLER, Princeton University, Princeton, NJ
VICKI L. CHANDLER, Gordon and Betty Moore Foundation, Palo Alto, CA
SEAN EDDY, HHMI Janelia Farm Research Campus, Ashburn, VA
MARK D. FITZSIMMONS, John D. and Catherine T. MacArthur Foundation, Chicago, IL
DAVID R. FRANZ, Midwest Research Institute, Frederick, MD
LOUIS J. GROSS, University of Tennessee, Knoxville, TN
JO HANDELSMAN, Yale University, New Haven, CT
CATO T. LAURENCIN, University of Connecticut Health Center, Farmington, CT
JONATHAN D. MORENO, University of Pennsylvania, Philadelphia, PA
ROBERT M. NEREM, Georgia Institute of Technology, Atlanta, GA
CAMILLE PARMESAN, University of Texas, Austin, TX
MURIEL E. POSTON, Skidmore College, Saratoga Springs, NY
ALLISON G. POWER, Cornell University, Ithaca, NY
BRUCE W. STILLMAN, Cold Spring Harbor Laboratory, Cold Spring Harbor, NY
CYNTHIA WOLBERGER, Johns Hopkins University School of Medicine, Baltimore, MD
MARY WOOLLEY, Research!America, Alexandria, VA

Staff

FRANCES E. SHARPLES, Director
JO L. HUSBANDS, Scholar/Senior Project Director
ADAM P. FAGEN, Senior Program Officer
MARILEE K. SHELTON-DAVENPORT, Senior Program Officer
INDIA HOOK-BARNARD, Program Officer
ANNA FARRAR, Financial Associate
CARL-GUSTAV ANDERSON, Senior Program Assistant
AMANDA P. CLINE, Senior Program Assistant
REBECCA L. WALTER, Senior Program Assistant
AMANDA L. MAZZAWI, Program Assistant

PREFACE

The US Department of Defense (DOD) is developing new efforts to protect warfighters from disease and biologic-warfare agents. The DOD Transformational Medical Technologies Initiative (TMTI) seeks to shorten the timeline for development of medical measures to counter emerging biologic-warfare threats: genetically engineered and other nontraditional toxins, virulence factors, and microorganisms. One goal of the TMTI is development of platforms for identifying unknown agents and developing countermeasures so that within five years an infrastructure will be in place for reacting quickly to a variety of threats, including agents that have been genetically engineered.

In response to a request from the Office of the Secretary of Defense, the National Academies formed the Standing Committee on Biodefense at the US Department of Defense. One purpose of the standing committee is to convene periodic meetings to discuss potential avenues for research, development, demonstration, and practical operational implementation of DOD's biologic-defense programs. Another purpose is to develop and coordinate studies and other activities in this field at the National Academies. On September 15, 2008, the National Academies held the workshop "Considerations for Ensuring Safety and Efficacy of Vaccines and Therapeutic Proteins Manufactured by Using Platform Approaches". The workshop was planned and organized by an ad hoc planning committee made up of members of the standing committee. The charge to the planning committee (see Appendix A) was to bring together scientists from academe, government, and the biotechnology industry to identify and discuss challenges and ideas related to the TMTI's vision of developing countermeasures within a few months after an agent is identified. The workshop focused (see Appendix B for agenda) on manufacturing processes and specifically on the development of "manufacturing platforms"— repeatable components of manufacturing that reduce both development time and risk. An underlying assumption was that demonstrating that integrated platforms can reliably produce safe and efficacious countermeasures might shorten the regulatory approval process.

Participants discussed manufacturing-related characteristics of monoclonal antibodies and vaccines. Although the planning committee understood that the TMTI efforts are broader than biologics and that TMTI platform approaches for biologics extend beyond monoclonal antibodies and vaccines, the planning committee believed that focusing on monoclonal antibodies and vaccines could illustrate some of the promise and challenges of platform approaches.

This summary is based on a transcript of the workshop, and statements are attributed to specific participants according to the transcript. It is presented as a narrative rather than a strict chronology to highlight the major themes that emerged from the meeting. Views expressed in the summary are those of the individual participants and are not necessarily those of the planning committee, the National Academies, or the project sponsor.

Jennie Hunter-Cevera, Chair
Planning Group for the Workshop on Considerations for Ensuring Safety and Efficacy of Vaccines and Therapeutic Proteins Manufactured by Using Platform Approaches

ACKNOWLEDGMENTS

The committee thanks those who made this workshop possible through their participation—speakers and panelists (their names and biographies are available in Appendix C) and the other workshop attendees. The workshop was successful in large part owing to the advance work conducted by the workshop planning group: Jennie Hunter-Cevera, Edward J. Arcuri, Stephen W. Drew, and Peter A. Patriarca. In accordance with National Research Council policies, the workshop planners were not involved in the preparation of this summary. James A. Marks, a member of the standing committee, provided insightful comments on early drafts of the summary.

This report has been reviewed in draft form by individuals chosen for their diverse perspectives and technical expertise, in accordance with procedures approved by the National Research Council's Report Review Committee. The purpose of this independent review is to provide candid and critical comments that will assist the institution in making its published workshop summary as sound as possible and to ensure that it meets institutional standards of objectivity, evidence, and responsiveness to the charge. The review comments and the draft manuscript remain confidential to protect the integrity of the deliberative process. We wish to thank the following individuals for their review of this summary:

L. Garry Adams, Texas A&M University
Jonathan Coffman, Wyeth BioPharma
Peter A. Patriarca, Biologics Consulting Group, Inc.

Although the reviewers and Dr. Marks have provided many constructive comments and suggestions, they were not asked to endorse the content nor did they see a final draft of the summary before its release. The review of this summary was overseen by **P. Frederick Sparling**, University of North Carolina. Appointed by the National Research Council, he was responsible for making certain that an independent examination of this summary was carried out in accordance with institutional procedures and that all review comments were carefully considered. Responsibility for the final content of this summary rests entirely with the institution.

CONTENTS

INTRODUCTION

A major goal of the US Department of Defense (DOD) Transformational Medical Technologies Initiative (TMTI) is to develop countermeasures that will protect military personnel against bioweapons, including specific infectious-disease agents and toxins. An explicit TMTI objective is to respond quickly to such threats by producing an appropriate amount of an effective countermeasure—currently defined as enough material to treat or vaccinate 3 million personnel—within 12 months of identification of a specific threat. DOD officials call for TMTI programs to be up and running by 2014. Whether countermeasure development and production capacity will be situated directly in DOD, solely in the private sector, or jointly in DOD and the private sector remains to be determined.

Achieving the goal may depend in large part on the availability of "manufacturing platforms" that are flexible and robust—capable of producing required quantities of finished products and capable of being redirected to make other products that address a particular threat. The requirements are all the more challenging because DOD has specified that countermeasures produced under the TMTI be reviewed and licensed by the Food and Drug Administration (FDA) before being deployed. Thus, an additional goal in identifying appropriate manufacturing platforms is to ensure that they can produce countermeasures that fulfill FDA criteria of safety and efficacy. It will also be necessary to identify the FDA review process that is best suited to such countermeasures, many of which would not be eligible for conventional clinical trials even if circumstances did not require accelerated review.

The condensed timetable that is intrinsic to the TMTI program will probably require that countermeasures being produced under its aegis be put on a regulatory fast track. Because many of the pathogens that are likely to be used as bioweapons are highly lethal, the FDA "animal rule" comes into play in evaluating the efficacy of novel countermeasures because their efficacy cannot be evaluated in clinical trials. However, such candidate countermeasures may still be subject to safety testing in clinical settings. The TMTI's condensed timetable is likely to drive countermeasure developers to pursue regulatory review at the same time as product-development efforts that include scaling up production.

With respect to the likely review of TMTI countermeasures, it is instructive to look at how FDA officials annually evaluate changes in the trivalent influenza vaccine, which is reformulated to optimize activity against currently circulating variants of the influenza virus. The vaccine is reformulated each year, but consistency in the manufacturing platform and the cumulative experience in producing and using the vaccine over several decades make it possible to review and approve each set of reformulated products rapidly—typically within 30 days. However, as discussed later in this summary, there may be limitations on the precedent set by the influenza example.[1]

[1]Another potential precedent, the European Union's so-called mockup vaccine dossiers for pandemic influenza vaccines, was noted during review. A regulatory authority essentially "preapproves" a pandemic vaccine on the basis of information provided on a surrogate influenza strain.

The TMTI is focusing on several classes of countermeasures. Low-molecular-weight drugs[2] make up one class, but biologics were the topic of this workshop. In particular, the workshop focused on therapeutic proteins in the form of monoclonal antibodies (MAbs) and on vaccines, whose principal role is to prevent infectious diseases. Both classes are capable of blocking the action of toxins that may be associated with infectious agents. MAbs were selected for discussion because of industry experience in manufacturing them with a platform approach. Although MAb production is by no means simple, industry representatives say that procedures for making such proteins and then scaling up their production are relatively routine and reliable. Vaccines were selected for discussion because their development is less straightforward. There is less uniformity because of the wide array of vaccine types, including live attenuated or killed viruses, killed bacterial cells, purified polysaccharides and proteins, glycoproteins, conjugate molecules, and vaccines that consist of DNA molecules that encode specific proteins.

TMTI Case For Versatile Production Platforms

Brian Reinhardt, TMTI discovery deputy, and Darrell Galloway, director of the Defense Threat Reduction Agency Chemical and Biological Technologies Directorate, described a key goal of the TMTI program as fostering development and production of broad-spectrum countermeasures against genetically modified and other novel biological threats. In the face of a threat, it will be critical to have available adequate amounts of appropriate countermeasures for protecting or treating US troops. To develop particular countermeasures, Galloway stated, it is essential first to identify the threat agents that might be or are being deployed. During the preliminary threat-identification phase, the TMTI envisions taking advantage of analytic platforms in several DOD programs, particularly the DNA-sequencing and bioinformatics capabilities in the US Army Medical Research Institute for Infectious Diseases at Fort Detrick in Frederick, Maryland. Some threat agents may consist of familiar biologic pathogens; others might be novel or "unknown"—consisting, for example, of components derived from two or more microbiologic pathogens or of components that are genetically engineered for novelty.

Galloway explained that the next stage of the countermeasure-development process, drug discovery, depends in part on identifying appropriate molecular targets in the threat agents and on finding appropriate chemical entities that can neutralize or inactivate them. This process will entail both analytic and empirical steps, including computer modeling, to determine which countermeasures are likely to be suitable for the particular threat agent at hand.

The TMTI expects that the countermeasures themselves will be produced to meet FDA good-manufacturing-practice standards and that enough will be produced at appropriate dosages to treat or to vaccinate several million US troops. (In some cases, that figure was presented as 3 million doses; in others, TMTI representatives mentioned producing quantities that could be used to treat 300,000 US troops. Dosing requirements

---

[2]Small molecules that can be synthesized chemically.

are uncertain because in some cases people might be treated with multiple doses of a vaccine or therapeutic product. Furthermore, the use of adjuvants with vaccines can allow lower doses.)

Those figures are tentative and subject to refinement, according to Galloway. In part, they are from figures developed through a separate program in the DOD Defense Advanced Research Projects Agency (DARPA), which specifies a timeline of 12 weeks for producing enough of a specific countermeasure to treat 3 million people. That DARPA program is exploring characteristics of rapid countermeasure production and has been focusing on plants, fungi, and bacteria as means for producing countermeasures.

Discussion Of TMTI Efforts

In discussion, Galloway said that one TMTI scenario is a single countermeasure-production facility with the capacity to produce appropriate quantities of 5 to 10 molecular entities per year; they could include MAbs, vaccines, and low-molecular-weight therapeutics. Such a facility could cost a few hundred million dollars to build and substantial amounts to maintain; therefore, the TMTI is analyzing alternatives before committing to that scenario. He also described the countermeasure capabilities in the TMTI as including some 40 separate projects, some of which operate with great rapidity. One goal is to integrate the separate projects to enable them to operate more efficiently in the overall countermeasure-discovery process. Galloway said that DOD expects some products to be produced and then stored and anticipates that some of these products will have shelf-lives of many years. There was some debate among workshop participants about whether products needed to be stable for many years and whether, instead of storing products for many years, robust production technologies could be used to meet supply demands on short notice, perhaps by holding appropriate precursors in storage so that they are ready for rapid end-product manufacture.

Some participants suggested that the latter approach provides an advantage—instead of relying on stored products, the TMTI program could specify short-term production of an alternative, possibly upgraded countermeasure, allowing for adjustments that take into account recent technical or scientific advances—and likened the adjustments to what happens each year when the seasonal influenza vaccine is produced.

However, Harry Greenberg, senior associate dean for research at Stanford University, said that the analogy does not fit the situation that the TMTI faces in that experience with the influenza vaccines covers at least 40 years of regular use in human populations, whereas the substitution of a new countermeasure for one that is only slightly older could not have built up a comparable clinical record. Other participants, such as Edward Arcuri, chief operating officer for VaxInnate[3], said that FDA officials are likely to scrutinize novel products derived from novel technologies more closely than products or processes that are considered proven and with which they have established "comfort levels". Similarly, David Robinson, vice president for bioprocess research and development at Merck, said that there are slightly different issues to deal with in developing countermeasures against familiar pathogens as opposed to countermeasures that will need to

[3] Edward Arcuri is now at Novartis Vaccines and Diagnostics, Inc.

be both safe and effective against biothreat "unknowns". Furthermore, even in dealing with surrogate markers for familiar pathogens, it is important to understand their pathology. Stephen W. Drew, of Drew Solutions and Science Partners LLC, pointed to several issues that should be noted for further consideration: how to choose countermeasure discovery and production platform, how to integrate such platforms, how to assemble a cadre of people to use and maintain the platforms, and how to keep the people up to date so they are prepared when called on to adapt the platforms to new demands.

PLATFOMS FOR LARGE-SCALE MONOCLONAL ANTIBODY PRODUCTION

Brian Kelley, senior director of bioprocess development at Genentech, and Dane Zabriskie, vice president of process development at Amgen, described similar processes for producing MAbs on an industrial scale for human health applications. Kelley said that large-scale MAb production processes are consistent and reliable, so they are more likely than an altogether novel approach to be used for producing therapeutic materials to meet the timetable specified by DOD under the TMTI. Except for minor differences in detail, Zabriskie generally agreed with Kelley about the feasibility of using MAb production platforms. However, both raised questions about the efficacy of MAbs as countermeasures against pathogens used in bioweapons. The details of their presentations and the discussion that followed are described in the next few pages.

Presentation by Brian Kelley

Genentech produces five FDA-licensed recombinant MAbs in four US facilities and a fifth being built in Singapore. Operations in all five facilities are based on large-scale mammalian cell culture, as are those of other large-scale MAb manufacturers, according to Kelley. In all, FDA has licensed more than 30 MAbs for clinical applications. It is important to note that except for one product, marketed as Synagis (a MedImmune product to protect infants against respiratory syncytial virus), currently licensed MAbs are not used for treating infectious diseases. Instead, most licensed MAbs are aimed at mainly chronic diseases.

Kelley framed the TMTI challenge partly as requiring manufacturing capacity to produce one million doses of antibody in less than 1 year or, in other terms, to produce on a 1,000-kg scale. Adapting the process quickly to cease making one type of MAb and start making another remains challenging, but the scale of MAb production is no longer considered a limiting factor. Indeed, during the last five years, improvements in productivity, including modification of mammalian cells to yield high-titer MAbs and then refinement of later-stage processes to purify them with greater efficiency, were so successful that the overall commercial capacity for producing MAbs exceeds current demand.

The Genentech approach to producing MAbs depends on several key elements, including the use of well-defined Chinese hamster ovary (CHO) cells; defined and consistent growth media and other materials, such as formulation buffers; standardized analytic technologies; a consistent purification process; and cumulative experience in refining and working with the production platform. Typically, once a particular recombinant MAb can be produced stably in a newly re-engineered CHO cell line, seed cells are introduced into a bioreactor for a 12- to 14-day batch-production cycle during which the product titer rises to about 2 g/L. Production can then be scaled up. For example, a facility equipped with six 15-kL bioreactors could produce about 4 tons of MAb products per year, according to Kelley.

One key technical drawback with respect to meeting TMTI timetables is that it typically takes four months to transfect, adapt, and select a modified CHO-producer cell for each new MAb entering production. Moreover, it may take a month to build up the cell-production stock for full-scale use. More time may be needed on the front end to identify at the molecular level appropriate criteria for the particular MAb being produced. However, if the MAb is based on antibodies obtained from a human who survived exposure to a specific threat agent, it might be possible to speed up this early phase.

There are other technical issues to consider, including whether IgG1 effector functions are sought, in which case the MAb will not perform properly unless it is appropriately glycosylated (modified by the addition of carbohydrates), and whether a particular MAb, because of its genetic sequence, will be "humanized" and also optimized for affinity. Such refinements can add several months to the early phase of development during which cells are being optimized for production.

In general, according to Kelley, the overall time to develop and produce a MAb is 14 months if no time to optimize the cell lines or other components of the process are included. During this period, a producer would also need to be working with FDA officials for the purpose of evaluating and licensing the final product, and also for certifying the production process insofar as is necessary. Kelley stated, in part because of such regulatory issues, it seems preferable to keep to the current, fully vetted approach to producing MAbs instead of switching to an alternative process. He noted that one potential way to shorten the current production timeframe—applicable only to threat agents already identified—is to develop a series of CHO-producer lines that could be stored for production use when needed.

In the event of an emergency in which DOD requires a particular countermeasure for treating US troops, it could be difficult to build and bring on line a new manufacturing facility to meet TMTI requirements, according to Kelley. He argued that it seems better to have a production facility that is poised for what he and others call a warm start, that is, ready to begin producing specified MAbs as soon as appropriate seed cells are provided. Such a facility might be a dedicated DOD facility that is already up and running. Alternatively, TMTI, through its commercial partners, might draw on the excess production capacity that is now in place in the private sector. In a fast-start or emergency production scenario, it might be possible to use disposable bioreactors, which are now being designed in the 2,000-L range, according to Kelley.

Another potential drawback with respect to meeting TMTI goals, according to Kelley, is that, for these early developmental steps en route to producing MAb countermeasure products, specific vectors, media, and tailored host cells tend to be covered by patents and thus raise intellectual-property (IP) issues. However, he believes that forging partnership and licensure agreements could overcome many or all IP-related obstacles. A nontechnical issue to address is that a fully outfitted large-scale production facility typically can cost as much as $800 million to build—a figure that is considerably higher than those mentioned by the TMTI.

Kelley summed up his presentation by concluding that product finish-and-fill issues and stability and safety questions pose fewer challenges than does the central question of determining the efficacy of MAbs that are produced as countermeasures against bioweapons. Assuming that phase 1 clinical-safety studies are required to satisfy FDA regulatory review, it could prove challenging to complete them within the specified product-delivery time; subjecting an MAb that targets an infectious agent to regulatory review by FDA as a test case would be a valuable exercise for determining how to approach that hurdle in the event of a genuine emergency. Kelley suggested that the public–private partnership forged during World War II to produce penicillin might be a useful model for the TMTI to consider.

Presentation by Dane Zabriskie

Amgen has four major manufacturing facilities, each equipped to produce MAbs on a 15-kL scale, and the company product pipeline includes more than 60 candidates, many of them MAbs, according to Zabriskie. The average time from gene construction to receipt of an investigational new drug (IND) approval for a MAb is 12–18 months.

Zabriskie pointed out that several features of Amgen's approach to selecting and producing MAbs are distinct from Genentech's and might help to accelerate production. For example, Amgen uses a "XenoMouse" in which the murine genes involved in antibody synthesis have been replaced with their human counterparts, so the antibodies produced are fully human rather than murine. Moreover, the company uses high-throughput robotic procedures to identify MAb-producing cells that will work with high efficiencies in later bioreactor steps.

Although the largest known bioreactor for growth of mammalian cell lines is thought to be the 25-kL vessel at Genentech, Zabriskie predicts that efficiency gains at the cell level and at other stages of MAb production between now and 2014 could mean that smaller bioreactors will be sufficient to meet TMTI-specified production goals. The overall yield of 10 MAbs that Amgen had in development as of 2005 varied from 40% to 80%; it was about 70% for most of them. When the process is scaled up to use 15-kL bioreactors, recovery is as high as 80%, for a yield of 4 g/L. Production efficiencies are improving; the cost of finished MAbs continues to drop and is expected to fall below $1,000/g soon, and with the cost of building a production facility with four 15-kL bioreactors and other equipment needed for finish-and-fill of final products about $1.8 billion—higher than some estimates.

Several steps in the production of clinically useful MAbs are considered routine by those working in this field, but technical challenges are expected to arise for each new product, according to Zabriskie. That expectation reflects the intrinsic heterogeneity and complexity of such molecules. For instance, the behavior of MAb proteins on cation-exchange columns, although often tractable, can prove unpredictable, reflecting heterogeneity in the surface charges of some of the proteins. Other sources of heterogeneity—including additions of sugars, oxidation, and deamidation of various amino acid side chains—change physical properties and could affect safety and efficacy. Product sponsors may be required to address such issues.

FDA officials routinely consider some 30 attributes of MAbs in their regulatory evaluations and for continuing quality-control purposes to characterize product lots for consistency after licensing. Zabriskie noted that stakeholders are working with FDA to establish acceptable critical quality attributes (CQAs) for raw materials and for process characteristics that could help sponsors and regulatory officials when they are using risk-management tools. FDA defines CQAs as factors that could affect the safety or efficacy of a biologic product; translating this broad definition into specific examples is a major challenge now facing the industry. For MAbs in particular, companies are determining whether minor changes meet the CQA threshold or are incidental to product safety and efficacy.

The 12- to 18-month timeline cited by Zabriskie starts with gene construction and ends with IND approval. In contrast, the overall development time from initial discovery to approval and manufacture of a therapeutic product ranges from 10 to 15 years, according to Zabriskie. The first seven years focus on in vitro and in vivo preclinical development and formulation of a product, including initial safety assessments. The next eight-year phase depends in large part on clinical development and evaluation and is very much "clinically driven." If TMTI products will not be subjected to traditional clinical-efficacy trials, the required safety and pharmacokinetic clinical trials could be completed in 7–12 months, according to Zabriskie. Nevertheless, determining the appropriate molecular targets for effective use of MAbs as countermeasures against particular biothreat agents is a time-consuming step—one that could take up to six years to complete, according to Zabriskie.

Zabriskie offered several recommendations:

- Work closely with FDA to determine whether a clinical-safety platform could be established that would apply broadly to countermeasures being developed.
- Focus attention on the drug-discovery process to make it faster and better able to predict the efficacy of novel countermeasures in humans.
- Accelerate the development of MAb cell lines to take less than the usual 6–12 months.
- Validate process platforms.
- Determine how to accept CQAs for MAbs as a class instead of case by case.
- Reframe the regulatory process for MAbs for DOD-related products to take into account the special circumstances surrounding biodefense situations.

Zabriskie framed the overall analysis of MAb readiness for the TMTI as a series of 10 critical readiness issues. He was optimistic about whether the platforms can produce most of the antibodies of interest; about the ability of platforms to lower costs of development, scale up and operation, and construction; and about the existence of a "common logic" in the industry. He was skeptical about whether CQAs can alone define safety and efficacy, saying that identification of a new regulatory approach for biodefense MAbs is most important. His outlook on the idea of producing supplies in 7–12 months is somewhere in the middle: have an early product serve as a surrogate for others and gain earlier FDA approval by using platforms.

Discussion

The workshop participants discussed whether it was reasonable to expect MAb production to supply TMTI-estimated needs, how to increase efficiency and reduce the timeline for producing necessary product, and industry versus government manufacturing facilities and the impact of issues beyond mere production capability.

Suitability of Platforms and Supply Needed

MAb production platforms appear suitable for supplying TMTI-estimated needed quantities of MAbs, according to Phil Gomez, of PRTM. Nonetheless, he recommended that the capacity issue be refined in terms of estimated doses that will be required to treat affected US forces. For instance, despite references to producing 1 million doses, enough to supply 1 g/soldier, it might be more realistic to speak in terms of milligrams per dose of some products. Participants noted that overall efficiencies might rise if effective doses were lower than the original assumption. Mark Schenerman, vice president of analytic biochemistry at MedImmune, said that that will affect planning for production facilities and manufacturing capacity and that product requirements might be reduced further if a product is packaged and stored in disposable units. However, he also noted that refining dose requirements would depend on what soldiers were exposed to.

Reducing Timeline

After discussing overall capability, workshop participants reviewed options for reducing timelines during the early phase of manufacturing. One approach would be to set up pools of cloned cells (a mixed population of cells, all producing the same antibody) at the early phase in which CHO cells are transfected with DNA that specifies which MAbs the cells are to make. Establishing pools of such cells might allow for selection of particular producer cells of higher efficiencies, and that choice might speed the overall production process. Jonathan Coffman, of Wyeth BioPharma, suggested that such a scenario may result in the manufacturing of 100,000 doses within about 100 days of the initial CHO-cell transfection. One idea raised was the use of "transient" transfectant cells to speed early steps toward production. A drawback to that approach is that such cells tend to be unstable; this is why they are used at Genentech for research and development but not for production, according to Kelley.

Zabriskie suggested a situation in which several MAbs against several potential pathogen targets could be made simultaneously and assessed in combination during the early phase of development, whereas selection for the most appropriate MAb in the mix would be delayed until much later in product development. In another option to cut time, Kelley said that MAb-producing cells that target known pathogens could be produced and banked for later use in the case of an emergency in which one or more of the specific pathogens were being deployed against US troops.

Most of the discussion centered around using mammalian cells to produce MAbs, but the group also discussed whether production timelines could be condensed by producing MAb molecules from *Escherichia coli* cells—a process that can speed production compared with the use of mammalian cells. Amgen has developed a "peptibody" product platform that combines a ligand-binding domain with the Fc domain of an antibody. The antibody-like products are produced in *E. coli*, according to Zabriskie. However, Kelley said that overall time savings through use of bacterial cells or similar alternative production sources are unpredictable, particularly because current purification procedures were developed on the basis of making MAbs in mammalian cells. In addition, bacterially produced MAbs would lack effector functions. In connection with the previous discussion of nonmammalian-cell platforms for producing MAbs, Greenberg said that FDA has dealt with about 30 MAb products that were produced from mammalian cells. The cumulative experience makes this platform attractive regardless of alternative approaches that depend on bacterial or other cells and that might speed some phases of the production process.

Placing the discussion of mammalian cell efficiencies in perspective, Kelley estimated that time savings from implementing even several of the refinements would be around 10–20%, not 50%, for overall production of MAbs.

Manufacturing Production Capacity

Moving beyond the discussion of whether MAb platforms in general are capable of meeting the TMTI's needs, participants discussed manufacturing facilities. Several discussed the pros and cons of the government's building its own countermeasure-production facility, which might be used by industry when it is not needed for TMTI production purposes, as opposed to leasing space in privately owned facilities. Participants discussed the merits of having a specialized MAb-production facility poised for action—what some called the warm-start option. In particular, Coffman pointed out that it would be helpful to have a team of skilled producers on hand who could keep in practice, perhaps by making about five MAb products per year. Gomez said that building a small, more flexible facility might be a way to give DOD experience in making a variety of countermeasure products.

Michael Ascher, of the University of California, Davis, and other participants asked whether industry could reserve MAb-production capacity for the TMTI to use in emergencies—for example, by maintaining extra capacity that would be kept "in tune" or up to date through intermittent use. Kelley and Zabriskie said that companies already have excess production capacity that could be drawn on as needed in a national emergency. To prepare for such emergencies, a participant suggested that the federal government should consider forming partnerships with companies and begin producing MAbs that target known pathogens as part of a preparedness exercise. Such partnerships and production runs could also be used to train personnel, providing them with the skills needed to conduct such large-scale, specialized production operations.

Regulatory Issues

The group discussed what Peter A. Patriarca, of Biologics Consulting Group, Inc., described as generally more time-consuming than production: consideration of safety and efficacy. Because postproduction regulatory issues might slow the approval process for countermeasures that the TMTI is seeking, several participants suggested that DOD consider investing in research that addresses the CQA issues outlined by Zabriskie above. Participants also noted that the FDA sponsors workshops that include exercises in which product sponsors submit mock IND filings to the agency as a way of gaining experience that can be used in shepherding real products through regulatory reviews. Specific safety and efficacy issues discussed are highlighted here.

Safety

Participants described regulatory consideration of MAb safety. Specifically, Zabriskie noted that the regulatory agencies focus on rare adverse events and on safety issues of theoretical concern in addition to the conventional ones, and Coffman pointed out that in his experience MAbs directed against human antigens fail safety and toxicity tests in about one-fourth of the cases. MAbs directed against nonhuman, nonanimal targets are less likely to have toxic side effects, although some tissue cross-reactivity can occur. Coffman suggested that DOD set up toxicology testing facilities to test any product quickly. Tissue cross-reactivity studies could also focus on antigens often seen in autoimmune disorders. A few specific types of possible risks posed by MAbs[4] were mentioned, but overall the discussions focused on how to make the consideration of risk efficient and appropriate.

Galloway noted that the DOD mandate for the TMTI calls for providing medical countermeasures for use by the "war-fighting community", not the general public. Such circumscribed use could influence decision-making about the safety of such products. Griffin Trotter, of Saint Louis University Center for Health Care Ethics, said that risk profiles of products should reflect whether soldiers need the countermeasures for an actual attack or need them for the possibility of a future attack. Leslie Benet, of the University of California, San Francisco, and other participants said that political pressure should be applied to FDA to ensure that development of MAb countermeasures has "no-fault" status. Other participants suggested that DOD make its case to FDA by presenting an analysis that emphasizes the value and benefit of such products over the risks that they pose. Robinson said that establishing a standard risk-benefit ratio for countermeasures would be helpful, but whether products for DOD could be held to different standards than those produced for the general population is a tricky issue, in part because of liability questions but also because of the possibility that negative publicity of any kind could damage corporate reputations.

Zabriskie said it would be helpful if FDA would serve as a forum for exchanging otherwise proprietary information about experiences with MAbs and vaccines, and thus for developing a better and shared understanding of "best practices" within these industry subspecialties. Fred Murphy, of the University of Texas Medical Branch at Galveston,

---

[4]MAbs directed against human targets, potential cross-reactions if soldiers receive both prophylactic vaccines and post-exposure therapy.

suggested that DOD, the National Institutes of Health, and the Centers for Disease Control and Prevention could also be involved in providing such a forum.

Efficacy

Although safety is important, the major issue concerning MAbs is efficacy, according to Zabriskie. Indeed, Ascher said that MAbs, when tested, have failed as potential countermeasures against several pathogens that might be used in bioweapons. MAbs were selected as a main subject of this workshop not because of their potential efficacy but because their production in a platform process is relatively well worked out. When the value of using MAbs as countermeasures against exotic, unknown, or synthetic pathogens was questioned, Galloway noted that TMTI and other agencies of the federal government are looking at many platforms and products to produce effective countermeasures.

Denise Faustman, of Harvard Medical School, and James A. Marks, of the University of California, San Francisco, raised the possibility of using polyclonal instead of monoclonal antibodies for counteracting pathogens. However, that approach could complicate regulatory reviews, particularly if a bank of several dozen MAb-producing cell lines were used to make the polyclonal-antibody mixture, according to Kelley.

PLATFORMS FOR VACCINE PRODUCTION

Presentation By David Robinson

Merck has been producing vaccines for more than 100 years. There are many varieties of vaccines, and they now include attenuated or inactivated viruses and bacteria; subunits made of polysaccharides, recombinant subunits from protein conjugates, and virus-like particles; and antigen-encoding vaccines consisting of plasmid DNA or modified adenoviruses that depend on cells in hosts to generate appropriate immunogens. Other companies are developing a baculovirus-based platform for making vaccines.

Merck recently built a pilot plant that incorporates several vaccine-production platforms, including a newer yeast-cell–based production system that is used when necessary for making glycoprotein immunogens. Within that facility, two platform systems can be run simultaneously in separate suites, and it is also possible to switch relatively quickly from one operation to another in the same space.

No platform process can cover the whole array of vaccines, according to Robinson, but DNA vaccines can be made from a single platform, and they can be used for producing a wide array of immunogens. Merck has not proved the clinical efficacy of any DNA-based vaccine product, but other producers are reporting success with DNA-based vaccines, including one that protects horses against West Nile virus and another that can protect salmon against a viral disease.

Similarly, the array of adenovirus-based vaccines is amenable to platform production, and genetically modified adenoviruses can elicit both cell-based and humoral immune responses in human hosts, according to Robinson. He explained that one problem with an adenovirus-based approach to making vaccines is that many humans are already exposed to serotype 5 of the adenovirus that is used for vaccines, so they are probably immune to the carrier virus and thus less susceptible to the sought-after vaccine responses. Again, as is the case with DNA-based vaccines, the clinical efficacy of adenovirus-based vaccines remains elusive. Indeed, Robinson stated that in a recent clinical study, recipients who had pre-existing immune responses to the adenovirus serotype 5 backbone of an experimental adenovirus-based vaccine intended to protect against HIV had higher infection rates than did recipients in the control group—a finding that remains unexplained.

Robinson described the Merck human papilloma virus (HPV) vaccine (marketed as Gardasil) as consisting of four recombinant yeast-produced conjugate proteins that were derived from, and now protect recipients against, the main serotypes of HPV that are responsible for causing genital warts and cervical cancer. The vaccine is administered with an alum adjuvant. Each of the four proteins is made in the same way, but one is much less stable than the other three. Dealing with that instability proved challenging during vaccine development, and the challenge was met by developing a complex disassembly and reassembly scheme involving chemical reducing agents. In addressing TMTI requirements with this system, vaccine developers can expect to face similar stability challenges during the initial seven month product-development phase, according to Robinson. Merck is now in phase 2 clinical testing of a similar conjugate vaccine that is designed to protect against the bacterial pathogen *Staphylococcus aureus*; the same production platform was adapted to deal with immunogens derived from this bacterial pathogen.

Robinson stated that Merck is concerned with CQAs as they apply to its variety of vaccines, and its standard approach is to look directly at characteristic signs of safety and efficacy in vaccines that are under development. Bioassays for determining CQAs for specific vaccine products remain proprietary. One key element on which release of a batch of product rests is a favorable result of cell-culture assays that shows that a vaccine continues to affect relevant cells, according to Robinson. Ligand-binding tests are also used, but they have to be validated through comparisons with clinical performance and shown to distinguish between good and bad lots of vaccine.

Robinson summarized his presentation by indicating that vaccine technologies are generally amenable to platform production, but the variety of approaches to making vaccines dictates a number of production platforms. Determining which vaccine type will be best suited for protecting against a particular threat agent is not straightforward. In addition, demonstrating the efficacy of some of the versatile vaccine platforms, such as the DNA-based and adenovirus-based platforms, is apt to prove challenging. Vaccine developers are immersed in determining efficacy, but Robinson stated that they also need to be developing appropriate bioassays that will later be used as surrogate markers of clinical efficacy.

Discussion

Participants discussed platform technologies, manufacturing, and regulatory and efficacy issues.

Various Platforms

Arcuri and Drew agreed with Robinson that a single platform for vaccine production is not possible; Drew estimated that about six distinct vaccine-production platforms are necessary.

A number of participants expressed optimism about the DNA-based platform. One stated that the reproducibility of production of DNA-based vaccines and vaccines based on recombinant proteins was comparable with the reproducibility of MAb production. Robinson said that development of DNA-based vaccines tends to be much faster; that is, it is faster in producing an experimental product that encodes a new antigen and in readying the product for a clinical trial. Such products can be made quickly, whereas other types of vaccines cannot be made within the 7–12 months that the TMTI has specified. Gomez pointed to development of a particular experimental vaccine for H5N1 influenza that was ready for clinical evaluation in about 6 months.

Robinson pointed out that regardless of production platform, predicting timelines for overall vaccine development is challenging, if not impossible. He summarized several Merck experiences in which development of particular vaccines, such as the rotavirus and varicella virus vaccines, each took about 20 years, and development of the HPV vaccine took about 10 years. As for which platform (DNA-based or other) might be used to produce a countermeasure against a particular agent, Robinson said that although vaccine-production processes are generally understood, choosing a particular approach for developing a vaccine for a novel agent can be challenging. In general, platform-based production lowers costs, but some production options may still prove expensive.

Manufacturing Facilities

Participants addressed production capacity for vaccines. In contrast with the capacity to produce antibodies, the industry does not have excess capacity for producing vaccines, according to Arcuri and Robinson, particularly vaccines that consist of live attenuated viruses. Robinson thought that it would be helpful for the government to foster the development of surge capacity, possibly by guaranteeing markets for such products. Contract manufacturers could help in meeting vaccine-production needs, but building production capacity among producers of specialized vaccines seemed preferable to at least one participant. The construction of multipurpose vaccine facilities is feasible; Merck has a pilot vaccine facility that is capable of running different platforms, and its versatility encompasses several production platforms, including adenovirus, *E. coli*, yeast, and CHO cells. Shifting from one cell type to another can take place within days, and personnel running the Merck facility are trained to work with the variety of platforms available there.

In response to questions about the current vision of a government-owned countermeasure-production facility, Jerome Donlon said that it would probably be built to produce both vaccines and MAbs on well-understood platforms but also include additional production components that are under development. Kelley pointed out that a operations capable of producing 100-kg batches of MAbs would have little overlap with vaccine-production operations if the two platforms were set up in a single facility, and Coffman suggested that it would be more practical to design separate facilities for the two platforms because housing them together could lead to less efficient production of MAbs.

Regulatory Issues

At least one participant thought that platform reliability is likely to be a plus for vaccines in dealing with FDA reviews. This participant noted that gaining regulatory acceptance of novel approaches, such as one that depends on baculovirus for production, would prolong initial reviews of vaccines that were intended to serve as TMTI countermeasures. For example, the first reviews of DNA-based vaccines drew heightened scrutiny from FDA.

Participants discussed the evaluation of whether a vaccine provides protective immunity. Robinson said that animal models are useful in some cases, particularly when a bioassay is sought for use in releasing vaccine lots; in the absence of an animal model of a particular disease, however, developing such bioassays can be difficult. Participants discussed ways other than animal-model bioassays to evaluate vaccine effectiveness. Robinson thought that obtaining neutralizing antibodies (for use as a surrogate measure of immunity or in animal bioassays) would be especially challenging in the case of an unknown or newly emerging biothreat agent. Participants asked whether there are general rules for determining what protective immunity will depend on. Robinson responded that it seems that only in relatively rare cases—such as those involving the updated influenza, pneumococcal, and HPV vaccines—might there be consistency in predicting how vaccines will behave. Research and empirical analysis typically are needed when one is selecting appropriate antibodies, including antibodies that will be used as reagents in bioassays, according to Robinson.

Greenberg described the influenza-vaccine experience. Decades of experience in adjusting the influenza vaccine each season provide some confidence that raising antibodies to a newly circulating hemagglutinin determinant of that virus will protect against influenza infections. However, making such changes in reformulating the seasonal influenza vaccine is far from perfect, and this might account for some of the variation in the vaccine's performance from year to year.

Consideration of what could be learned from the influenza-vaccine experience led to questions about the role and value of vaccine adjuvants in recent efforts to expand coverage of the influenza vaccine. Greenberg said that adjuvants typically increase the quantitative, not the qualitative, immune response to a vaccine. However, by intensifying overall responses to a particular vaccine, an adjuvant might broaden coverage by raising host responses to ordinarily minor epitopes that might otherwise have remained undetected by the humoral components of the host immune system. Richard Jaffe, Senior Medical Advisor at the Office of the Deputy Assistant to the Secretary of Defense for Chemical and Biological Defense and Chemical Demilitarization Programs, said that something similar happens at the cellular level: a minor component of a pathogen may trigger an immune response in T cells.

The discussion shifted to the use of vaccines against intracellular bacterial pathogens and the pathogens that cause hemorrhagic fever; these pathogens are the subjects of TMTI efforts. Several participants stated that the development of vaccines to protect against intracellular pathogens remains particularly challenging, if not intractable. Galloway pointed out that the TMTI is not committed to developing conventional vaccines and is seeking novel ways to induce protective host responses.

SUMMARY OF KEY POINTS

Patriarca reviewed what was discussed at the workshop, namely the prospects of producing adequate supplies of safe and effective MAbs and vaccines to meet TMTI needs to provide US military forces with countermeasures against biothreats. Patriarca thought that, in general, it appears feasible to produce enough MAbs or vaccines within the TMTI-designated timeframe. However, he described several additional key points of the workshop:[5]

- *Manufacturing* of MAbs appears relatively straightforward, but it is not the most time-consuming step in the development of countermeasures, in his view. Participants urged further discussion of *discovery*-related issues for critical products.
- Vaccine-manufacturing platforms are considerably more complicated than those for MAbs; there are at least a half-dozen such platforms for making vaccines, and only some are well characterized. However, Jennie Hunter-Cevera[6], of the University of Maryland Biotechnology Institute, noted that discovering molecular targets, which is essential in developing MAbs, is not always needed for vaccine development.
- Demonstrating safety and efficacy of both vaccine-based and MAb-based countermeasures will be challenging even with the use of surrogate end points. As emphasized by Schenerman, it will be important to devise a risk–benefit algorithm to satisfy FDA criteria for evaluating the safety and efficacy of biothreat countermeasures for US troops in the face of an emergency.

[5]The summary statements made by Peter Patriarca reflect his views and are not meant to imply a consensus of the workshop participants.
[6]Jennie Hunter-Cevera is now at RTI International.

Appendix A

Statement of Task

An ad hoc committee will plan and conduct a public workshop that focuses on the manufacturing process and specifically on the development of "manufacturing platforms"—repeatable components of manufacturing that aim to reduce both development time and risk of vaccines and therapeutic proteins (e.g., monoclonal antibodies) targeted at specific agents within a few months after these agents are identified. This is important because a major component of the U.S. Department of Defense (DoD)/Transformational Medical Technologies Initiative (TMTI) efforts in biodefense is to develop vaccines and therapeutic proteins (e.g., monoclonal antibodies) targeted at specific agents within a few months after agents are identified. The workshop will feature invited presentations and discussions on various topics addressing integrated platforms to produce safe and efficacious surrogate countermeasures in contexts that are expected to mimic those of future threat agents and that could shorten the regulatory approval process. The agenda will include manufacturing-related characteristics of monoclonal antibodies and vaccines that confer safety and efficacy, attempting to highlight the most important critical quality attributes (CQAs) that stem from these characteristics and discussion of the extent to which these CQAs could form a basis for assuring production of safe and efficacious vaccines against novel agents, facilitating rapid approval of DoD countermeasure products by the FDA. It will also include the impact of the identified CQAs on the development/planning of manufacturing platforms and integration across multiple platforms, asking what should be considered in the development of manufacturing platforms to maximize the potential for consistency between existing and new monoclonal antibodies and vaccines. Additional discussion will center on whether there are characteristics of diseases or vaccines that will more readily lead to consistency between surrogate and new vaccines.

Appendix B

AGENDA

Considerations For Assuring Safety And Efficacy Of Vaccines And Therapeutic Proteins Manufactured Using Platform Approaches

September 15, 2008
National Academies Keck Center, Washington, DC

8:00 a.m. **Introduction to Workshop Objectives and Organizational Strategy**
Peter A. Patriarca, M.D.
Senior Clinical Consultant; Biologics Consulting Group, Inc.

8:15 **TMTI's Grand Vision/Premise for Developing Platforms to Manufacture and Develop Vaccines and Therapeutic Proteins**
Brian Reinhardt, TMTI Discovery Deputy

9:00 **Platforms for Rapid, Large-Scale Monoclonal Antibody Development & Production**
Brian Kelley. Ph.D.
Senior Director, Bioprocess Development, Genentech

9:30 Questions for Brian Kelley

10:00 Break

10:15 **Platform Technologies for the Development and Production of Monoclonal Antibody Biopharmaceuticals**
Dane Zabriskie, Ph.D.
Vice President, Global Process Development, Amgen Inc.

10:45 Questions for Dane Zabriskie

11:15 **What are General Guidelines or "Rules of Thumb" for Monoclonal Antibody Platforms? How Can These be Applied to TMTI Approaches?**

Discussion (led by Peter Patriarca)

- *TMTI*
- *Jonathan Coffman, Ph.D.; Wyeth BioPharma*
- *Phil Gomez, Ph.D., Principal, PRTM*
- *Mark A. Schenerman, Ph.D.; Vice President, Analytical Biochemistry, MedImmune*

12:45 Lunch

1:30 **Process Of Using Platform Approach To Facilitate FDA Approval: Insight From Merck Yeast Platform Products**
David K. Robinson, Ph.D.
VP BioProcess R&D, Merck & Co., West Point, PA.

2:00 Questions for David K. Robinson

2:30 **What are General Guidelines or "Rules of Thumb" for Manufacturing Using Yeast Platforms? How Can These be Applied to TMTI Approaches?**

Discussion (led by Peter Patriarca)

- *TMTI*
- *Jonathan Coffman, Ph.D.; Wyeth BioPharma*
- *Phil Gomez, Ph.D., Principal, PRTM*
- *Pascal Longchamp, Ph.D., MBA; VP of Business Development, Evolva*
- *Mark A. Schenerman, Ph.D.; Vice President, Analytical Biochemistry, MedImmune*

3:15 **Discussion of Questions Prepared by Committee**
Peter Patriarca

4:00 Break

4:15 **Continued Discussion of Questions Prepared by Committee**

5:15 **Summary's of Today's Themes**
Peter Patriarca

5:30 **Adjourn**

Appendix C

Biographies[7]

Planning Committee Members:

Jennie Hunter-Cevera, PhD (Chair) serves as president of the University of Maryland (MD) Biotechnology Institute. Previously, she had been the director of the Center for Environmental Biotechnology at the E. O. Lawrence Berkeley National Laboratory. She cofounded two small companies that did contract work for large pharmaceutical and biotechnology companies, consulted in a variety of biotechnology fields, and worked at Cetus Corporation and E. R. Squibb and Sons. She served as president of the Society of Industrial Microbiology (SIM), the United States Federation for Culture Collections (USFCC), and the International Marine Biotechnology Association. She served as senior editor of the *Journal of Industrial Microbiology*. Dr. Hunter-Cevera also served as a member of US Department of Agriculture Secretary Glickman's Genetic Resources Advisory Board and President Clinton's Department of State Council on Genetically Modified Foods. She served as the US representative to the Organisation for Economic Co-operation and Development on biological resource centers. Dr. Hunter-Cevera was elected to the American Academy of Microbiology, was elected a SIM Fellow in 1997, and received the SIM Charles Porter Award and the USFCC/J. Roger Porter Award (in recognition of her expertise in microbial cultures). She has been recognized as one of MD's Top 100 Women and one of the 50 Most Influential People in MD. Dr. Hunter-Cevera served on Governor Ehrlich's Technology Commission and the Governor's Executive Council for Transition, and chairs the MD Technology Development Corporation Board of Directors. She is a member of the Entremed Board of Directors, the MD Industrial Partnerships, the BioIT Coalition, MDBio, the MD Israeli Development Corporation, and the Center for Emerging Technologies. She also chairs SIM's Committee on Public Responsibility and Policy. Dr. Hunter-Cevera holds several patents on natural products and enzymes and has written many scientific publications in microbial ecology and screening. She has chaired two National Research Council committees.

Edward Arcuri, PhD, is the chief operating officer for VaxInnate, which he joined in June 2007. VaxInnate works to produce novel vaccines for seasonal and pandemic influenza. Dr. Arcuri has expertise in developing vaccines, including completing Food and Drug Administration approval and managing large-scale manufacturing. Previously, he was at Emergent BioSolutions, Inc., where he served as chief operating officer and was directly responsible for all development, manufacturing, and project-management activities. Before his position at Emergent, Dr. Arcuri held executive positions at MedImmune, Inc. where he was instrumental in the manufacture of Synagis, a treatment for respiratory syncytial virus, and FluMist, for protection against viral influenza. He has

[7] Affiliations at time of workshop are described in this appendix.

held a variety of executive, scientific, and research positions at Aviron, Inc., North American Vaccine, Inc., SmithKline Beecham, Merck & Co., The Helicon Foundation, and Oak Ridge National Laboratory. Dr. Arcuri graduated with honors with a degree in Biology from the State University of New York at Albany and went on to earn his MS and PhD in biology from Rensselaer Polytechnic Institute.

Stephen W. Drew (NAE), PhD, is a former Distinguished Senior Scientist at Merck & Co., Inc., where his responsibilities encompassed technology transfer and the development of new process technologies for pharmaceutical manufacturing. He has now started two companies: Drew Solutions LLC, a direct-consulting company (sole proprietor), and Science Partners LLC, an advocacy company for medicines and technologies. In the Merck Manufacturing Division (MMD), he has been vice president of vaccine science and technology, vice president of vaccine operations, and vice president of technical operations and engineering. Before joining MMD in 1987, he was the senior director of biochemical engineering in the Merck Research Laboratories, a department that he started in 1981. At Merck, he contributed to the process development and manufacture of several conventional and recombinant microbial products, including antibiotics and vaccines. His contributions in synthetic chemistry include the development of several processes for products and intermediates manufactured worldwide. Dr. Drew has expertise in chemical, biologic, and engineering technology for bulk manufacture of pharmaceuticals; capital project engineering; process safety testing and engineering; process control systems; information systems; fermentation and isolation process engineering for injectable antibiotics; anthelmintics; growth permitants; human and animal vaccines, including recombinant biologics; automated fermentation analyses; process control strategies for chemical and biologic processes; nanotechnology, biotechnology, and chemistry; intelligence and threat analysis; sensor systems; and weapons. Dr. Drew received his BS (1967) and MS (1969) in food science from the University of Illinois and his PhD (1974) in biochemical engineering from the Massachusetts Institute of Technology (MIT). He was elected to NAE in 1993 and is a member of several professional organizations in chemical engineering, chemistry, and biology. He has held offices in the American Institute of Chemical Engineers, the American Chemical Society, the American Society for Microbiology, and the Society for Industrial Microbiology and is a Fellow of the American Institute for Medical and Biological Engineering. He has served as chairman of the advisory committee to the Engineering Directorate of the National Science Foundation and served on several of its panels and studies. He has also served the departments of chemical engineering of several universities as a member of review committees and the MIT Center for Biomedical Engineering, Biotechnology Process Engineering Center, and Division of Biological Engineering.

Peter A. Patriarca, MD, earned his BS at the University of Notre Dame and his MD at Tulane University School of Medicine and is a board-certified pediatrician. Dr. Patriarca served as a commissioned officer in the US Public Health Service from 1980 to 2000. During that time, he worked at the Food and Drug Administration (FDA), where he served as director of the Division of Viral Products in the Office of Vaccines Research. He also served as division director in the Center for Biologics Evaluation and Research, where he worked on quality and consistency of chemical-manufacturing controls and clinical reviews and was intimately involved with regulatory decisions and policy affecting the development and approval of numerous investigational products. At the Centers for Disease Control and Prevention, he was a field and clinical investigator, with about 100 peer-reviewed journal publications, and contributed to immunization programs and policy promulgated through the Advisory Committee on Immunization Practices. Dr. Patriarca's product experience includes vaccines, plasma derivatives, monoclonal antibodies, and small molecules. He has expertise in influenza, poliomyelitis, measles, and pertussis and extensive international experience, vaccine-policy experience, and experience as an investigator in epidemiologic research and large-scale vaccine-efficacy studies. Dr. Patriarca serves as senior clinical consultant for the Biologics Consulting Group, Inc., in Bethesda, MD, where he provides a wide range of regulatory advice to clients in the drug industry, focusing primarily on vaccines and other biologic products. Dr. Patriarca's specialties include regulatory strategy, product-development strategy, clinical-protocol design, and submission preparation and review. Before working for the Biologics Consulting Group, Inc., Dr. Patriarca was the corporate head and vice president of worldwide regulatory affairs and pharmacovigilance for MedImmune, Inc., from 2001 to 2005.

Speakers and Invited Discussants:

Brian Kelley, PhD, is the senior director of bioprocess development at Genentech, which is responsible for development, validation, and technology transfer of fermentation, cell-culture, chromatography, and filtration steps for the production of recombinant therapeutic proteins derived from mammalian and bacterial hosts. He joined Genentech in 2007 after working for 15 years at Genetics Institute. From 1992 to 2007, he served as an adjunct faculty member of the Chemical and Biological Engineering department at Tufts University, where he taught two graduate classes each year on principles of cell and microorganism cultivation and protein purification. He obtained his BS in chemical engineering from the University of Wisconsin-Madison, and his PhD from the Massachusetts Institute of Technology. His interests include experimental design and other statistical methods applied to process development, filtration for cell and virus removal, ultrafiltration of high-concentration protein solutions, development of novel affinity chromatography ligands for protein purification, and high-throughput chromatographic development. Dr. Kelley has been active in the American Chemical Society's Biotechnology Division, chairing sessions on biopharmaceutical-process validation since 1997. He is on the PDA Biotechnology Advisory Board and has chaired the Recovery of Biological Products Board.

David Robinson, PhD, is vice president for bioprocess research and development (BPR&D) at Merck and Co. In this position, he leads the area responsible for the clinical bulk-supply manufacturing and process, analytic, and formulation development of Merck's biologic programs—vaccines, therapeutic proteins, and follow-on biologics/Merck BioVentures. The area has supported programs that have led to the approval of over a dozen products, including Merck's cervical-cancer vaccine, Gardasil;

rotavirus vaccine, RotaTeq; and shingles vaccine, Zostavax. Dr. Robinson received his BS in chemical engineering from the University of California, Berkeley and his PhD in chemical engineering from the Massachusetts Institute of Technology. He served as a postdoctoral fellow at the ETH Zurich and held an adjunct faculty position for 10 years in the Columbia University Department of Chemical Engineering. After working for Sandoz in Switzerland and later in New Jersey, Dr. Robinson worked in basic research at Merck in the Cell and Molecular Biology Department in Rahway. He spent a year at Schering-Plough and returned to Merck in 1997 as director in BPR&D, leading the biocatalysis group. He was later senior director and then executive director of BPR&D, chair of the Technology Transfer Team, and cochair of the Project Team for the rotavirus vaccine.

Dane Zabriskie, PhD, is vice president of process development at Amgen, Inc. The process-development organization supports the design, startup, and licensure of new plants and products and ensures that Amgen's manufacturing processes consistently produce safe and effective products in an efficient manner. Dr. Zabriskie came to Amgen in January 2004 from Biogen, where he had worked since 1998, most recently as vice president of the process-development organization. At Biogen, he was responsible for physical product development, including cell-line development, process development and scaleup, pharmaceutical sciences, analytic development, and the preparation of CMC regulatory documents. Before joining Biogen, Dr. Zabriskie spent 14 years with the biopharmaceutical research and development unit of SmithKline Beecham, during which he chaired the Biological Weapons Convention Subcommittee for Pharmaceutical Research and Manufacturers of America. He also cofounded and worked for 5 years at a small biotechnology company and spent 3 years as an assistant professor of chemical engineering at the State University of New York at Buffalo. Dr. Zabriskie received his PhD in chemical and biochemical engineering from the University of Pennsylvania, and he has undergraduate degrees in biochemistry and chemical engineering from Princeton University. Dr. Zabriskie has led the development of more than 20 biopharmaceutical products, including recombinant vaccines, monoclonal antibodies, fusion proteins, and other therapeutic proteins and products from mammalian cell and microbial sources.

Leslie Z. Benet (IOM), PhD, is a professor and former chairman of the Department of Biopharmaceutical Sciences at the University of California, San Francisco. His research interests, over 480 publications, and 11 patents are in pharmacokinetics, biopharmaceutics, and pharmacodynamics. His most recent work has addressed the cooperative effects of metabolic enzymes and transport proteins as related to immunosuppressive, anticancer, anti-AIDS, cardiovascular, and antiparasitic drugs and drugs of importance to women's health. He is a Fellow of the American Association for the Advancement of Science, the American Association of Pharmaceutical Scientists (AAPS), and the Academy of Pharmaceutical Research and Science. He is the chairman of the board of AvMax, Inc., and serves as a consultant to several pharmaceutical and biotechnology companies. Dr. Benet is a recipient of the AAPS Distinguished Pharmaceutical Scientist Award, the American Pharmaceutical Association Higuchi Research Prize, the American Society for Clinical Pharmacology Rawls-Palmer Award for Progress in Medicine, the International Pharmaceutical Federation (FIP) Høst-Madsen Medal, the University of California, San Francisco Distinguished Clinical Research

Lectureship, and six honorary doctorates. He previously served as chair for the Food and Drug Administration (FDA) Center for Biologics and Research External Peer Review Committee, the FDA Expert Panel on Individual Bioequivalence, and the FIP Board of Pharmaceutical Sciences and as a member of the FDA Science Board and the Board of Directors of the Institute for One World Health and the Board of Directors of the American Foundation for Pharmaceutical Education . Dr. Benet has served as the chair or a member of various IOM committees; he is a member of the Forum on Drug Discovery, Development and Translation. He served as the chair of the National Academies committee that produced the report *Giving Full Measure to Countermeasures: Addressing Problems in the DoD Program to Develop Medical Countermeasures Against Biological Warfare Agents*.

Jonathan Coffman, PhD, is a laboratory head overseeing the development of downstream processes for protein therapeutics at Wyeth BioPharma. He has been responsible for the transfer of over ten molecules to downstream clinical manufacturing. His work has influenced the development of all the downstream processes of protein therapeutics developed at Wyeth over the last 5 years. He has been the Development Team leader coordinating the overall development and technology transfer for two clinical molecules. Dr. Coffman has made numerous contributions to the development and transfer of purification processes for manufacturing of biologic products, including Wyeth's platform two-column-antibody purification process, and the regular use of high-throughput screening in downstream process development. Dr. Coffman received a PhD in chemical engineering from the University of Wisconsin. He has served in various capacities in the American Chemical Society Division of Biochemical Technology: he has been 2003 division program cochair, division secretary in 2004–2006, and Web Seminar Program coordinator since 2005, and he has been named the 2010 cochair for recovery of biologic products. He received the James M. Van Lanen Distinguished Service Award from the division in 2008.

Philip E. Coyle III, MS, served as assistant secretary of defense and director of operational test and evaluation in the Department of Defense (DOD). In this capacity, he was the principal adviser to the secretary of defense and the under secretary of defense for acquisition, technology, and logistics on test and evaluation in DOD. Mr. Coyle has 30 years of experience in testing and test-related matters. From 1959 to 1979 and again from 1981 to 1993, he worked at the Lawrence Livermore National Laboratory in Livermore, California, where he served as an associate director. In the Carter administration, Mr. Coyle served as principal deputy assistant secretary for defense programs in the Department of Energy; he had oversight responsibility for the department's nuclear-weapons testing programs. The International Test and Evaluation Association awarded Mr. Coyle the Allan R. Matthews Award, its highest award, for his contributions to the management and technology of testing and evaluation. He was awarded the Defense Distinguished Service Medal by DOD Secretary Perry and the Bronze Palm of the Defense Distinguished Service Medal by Secretary Cohen. Mr. Coyle received an MS (1957) in mechanical engineering and a BA (1956) from Dartmouth College. He is now affiliated with Science Strategies.

Denise L. Faustman, MD, PhD, has worked in autoimmunity for over 15 years and has made some of the key discoveries regarding the role of MHC class I antigen presentation in immunity. Her earlier research achievements include introducing the concept of modifying antigens on donor tissues to prevent their rejection, which is now in clinical trials for diverse human diseases treatable with cellular transplantation. In 2001, her laboratory reversed type 1 diabetes in mice with end-stage disease, and this project is now being translated into clinical trials. Her current research continues to focus on uncovering new treatments for type 1 diabetes and to search for therapies for other autoimmune diseases, including Crohn disease, lupus, scleroderma, rheumatoid arthritis, Sjögren syndrome, and multiple sclerosis. Dr. Faustman is director of the Immunobiology Laboratory at the Massachusetts General Hospital (MGH) and an associate professor of medicine at Harvard Medical School. After completing her internship, residency, and fellowships in internal medicine and endocrinology at the MGH, Dr. Faustman became an independent investigator at the MGH and Harvard Medical School in 1987. She is a member of the American Association for the Advancement of Science and has served on IOM committees. In 2003, Dr Faustman was honored by the National Institutes of Health and the National Library of Medicine with the Changing the Face of Medicine Award. She was one of 300 American physicians honored for achievement in medicine, past and present. In 2005, she received the Oprah Achievement Award for Top Health Breakthrough by a Female Scientist. In 2006, she was awarded the Women in Science Award, given by the American Medical Women's Association and Wyeth Pharmaceutical Company to a female physician who has made exceptional contributions to medical science through basic-science publications and leadership in the field.

Phil Gomez, PhD, MBA, has more than 15 years of experience in bringing drugs and biologics to market, working in both industry and government. He joined PRTM Management Consultants from the Vaccine Research Center at the National Institute of Allergy and Infectious Diseases, where he established the Vaccine Production Program in 2001, growing it to over 150 staff and completing the 126,000-ft^2 Vaccine Pilot Plant. During his 6-year tenure at the National Institutes of health (NIH), his group manufactured over 40 bulk pharmaceutical compounds and more than 15 candidate vaccines using innovative collaborations with industry to forward the development of vaccines against HIV, Ebola virus, Marburg virus, West Nile virus, severe acute respiratory syndrome, and influenza. Before going to NIH, Dr. Gomez spent over 9 years at Abbott Laboratories, Sanofi Pasteur, and Baxter Healthcare in positions of increasing responsibility, leading process and product development organizations and project teams for multiple biologic products. Dr. Gomez received an AB from Dartmouth College, an MS and a PhD in chemical engineering from Lehigh University, and an MBA from the Smith School of Business at the University of MD. Dr. Gomez earned the NIH Director's Award in 2007 for the establishment of the Vaccine Pilot Plant and rapid production of a pandemic influenza vaccine.

Charles H. Hobbs, DVM, is the director of toxicology at the Lovelace Respiratory Research Institute. Dr. Hobbs's primary research interests are in the long-term biologic effects of inhaled materials and the mechanisms by which they occur. His experience covers inhaled nuclear and chemical toxicants and infectious diseases. His research has covered physical and chemical characterization of airborne toxicants, in vitro mechanistic and toxicologic studies and long-term studies in laboratory animals of the relationships between dose to critical tissues and resulting biologic effects, and the important mechanisms active in determining these relationships. Dr. Hobbs has also been heavily involved in research management. He has focused on the direction and use of multidisciplinary teams of personnel to address complex problems. Previously, he was associate director and assistant director of the Inhalation Toxicology Research Institute, and vice-president of Lovelace Biomedical and Environmental Research Institute. Before that, he took a leave of absence from the Lovelace Biomedical and Environmental Research Institute to be a scientist in the Division of Biomedical and Environmental Research of the US Energy Research and Development Administration, and he has worked as an assistant director and toxicologist at the Inhalation Toxicology Research Institute at the Lovelace Foundation for Medical Education and Research. Dr. Hobbs received his DVM in 1966 from the Colorado State University in Fort Collins and professional certifications in veterinary medicine from Colorado, Wyoming, and New Mexico. He became a diplomate of and received certification in general toxicology from the American Board of Veterinary Toxicology in 1972 and 1981, respectively.

Pascal Longchamp, PhD, MBA, leads the worldwide business effort of Evolva as vice president of business development. He holds a PhD in microbiology and genetics from the University of Lausanne and did postdoctoral studies at the University of California, Berkeley. He was then engaged in anthrax studies at Lawrence Berkeley National Laboratory before joining Maxygen Inc. in the Silicon Valley, where he was involved in the Defense Advanced Research Projects Agency's Unconventional Pathogen Countermeasure program. That exposure to the biodefense field raised his awareness of the potential threat of microorganisms. After leaving Maxygen Inc. to become director of business development at Phyllom, he obtained an MBA and joined Evolva, a young biotechnology company that had invented a technology for applying directed evolution principles to small molecules for the pharmaceutical industry. Soon after joining Evolva, Dr. Longchamp recognized the potential of the technology for the biodefense industry. After a successful application to the Transformational Medical Technologies Initiative of the Defense Threat Reduction Agency (DTRA), Evolva is now applying its novel drug-discovery engine to generate novel immunomodulators, antivirals, and antibacterials for DTRA.

James D. Marks (IOM), MD, PhD, is professor of anesthesia and pharmaceutical chemistry at the University of California, San Francisco. He is board-certified in internal medicine, anesthesia, and critical-care medicine. From 1996 to 2001, he was the medical director of the Medical-Surgical Intensive Care Unit at San Francisco General Hospital, and he continues to attend in the intensive-care unit and operating rooms there. Dr. Marks is a pioneer in antibody engineering, in which he has developed widely used technology for generating and optimizing human therapeutic antibodies. He directs a research group that is using antibody gene-diversity libraries and display technologies to dissect the molecular basis of infectious diseases and cancer and to develop novel antibody-based therapeutic approaches for these diseases. His research in oncology has elucidated the effects of antibody biophysical properties on tumor targeting, and his laboratory has generated a novel antibody-based drug that is being commercialized for breast-cancer therapy. His laboratory works to develop antibody-based therapies for the biothreat agent botulinum neurotoxin. Dr. Marks has served on Department of Health and Human Services and National Institute of Allergy and Infectious Diseases expert advisory panels on the botulinum neurotoxins. He has more than 110 publications in antibody engineering and is an inventor on 62 issued or pending patents. He was elected to IOM in 2006.

Mark Schenerman, PhD, is vice president for analytic biochemistry at MedImmune and is responsible for structural and biologic characterization of preclinical and clinical products, stability and release testing of clinical products, technology transfer to quality control, and continuing product-development support. Since joining MedImmune in 1994, Dr. Schenerman has played an integral role in developing the company's analytic biochemistry function, and he leads a team of more than 90 scientists supporting all stages of product development. Before joining the company, Dr. Schenerman held positions in biologics development and research and development at Bristol-Myers Squibb Company and as a postdoctoral associate at Cornell University. He earned his bachelor's degree in medical technology at the University of Maryland and his doctorate in biochemistry and molecular biology at the University of Florida.